The Really Useful Guide to Natural Health and Beauty

Catherine Beattie

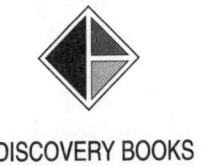

DISCOVERY BOOKS

First published in 1998 by Discovery Books
29 Hacketts Lane Pyrford Woking
Surrey GU22 8PP

© Catherine Beattie 1998

Catherine Beattie asserts the moral right to be
identified as the author of this work

*All rights reserved. No part of this publication may be
reproduced, stored in a retrieval system or
transmitted in any form or by any means, electronic,
mechanical, photocopied, recorded or otherwise,
without the prior permission in writing of Discovery
Books.*

A CIP catalogue record for this book is available
from the British Library
ISBN 0 9518511 9 5

Designed and typeset by David Simpson

Printed and bound in Great Britain by
Caledonian International Book Manufacturing Ltd,
Glasgow.

Contents

Acknowledgments 4

Introduction 5

Part One

    A Natural Alternative 7

    Therapies and Treatments 9

Part Two

    Symptoms and Health Conditions 43

Part Three

    Spa and Beauty Therapies 59

Part Four

    Registers and Association Addresses 75

Index 87

Acknowledgments

I would like to thank Joanna Pope, for her cheerful and invaluable help during all stages of researching and writing this book.

My warmest thanks to David Simpson for all his helpful advice and for designing the page layouts and alternative health symbols.

I should also like to thank the many associations, registers and practitioners of alternative medicine, who have furthered my understanding of the subject.

Finally, my special thanks to Alec for his continuous support, and to all my family for their interest and encouragement.

Introduction

The aim of this little book is to provide concise and practical information on two areas of natural health care currently enjoying a boom in popularity – alternative medicine and therapeutic spa and beauty treatments.

The first part of the book deals with alternative medicine, explaining what it is, how its philosophy differs from orthodox Western medicine and what to expect from your first consultation. A wide range of therapies and diagnostic techniques are described in detail.

Part Two looks at various symptoms and conditions that have responded to alternative health care, with details of helpful treatments and remedies.

Part Three – the spa and beauty section – describes the pampering therapies offered at spas, health resorts and beauty salons. It will help you decide what treatments to try when taking that revitalising break you've always promised yourself.

So that you can find out more about any of the treatments or therapies described, or the whereabouts of practitioners in your area, the final part of the guide includes an extensive list of alternative health associations, registers and other useful addresses and phone numbers.

Making that first call could be the start of a whole new approach to your health and lifestyle.

Advice to Readers

Always seek advice from your doctor if you are worried about any aspect of your health.

Consult your doctor about health symptoms *before* seeing an alternative practitioner.

Let your doctor know what alternative treatments you are having or intend to try.

Inform your alternative practitioner about your conventional treatments and prescribed medications.

Research is ongoing to establish the health claims of many of the therapies and treatments described in this book. Alternative health care is not based on scientific fact, nor has its effectiveness been subjected to the same critical scrutiny as orthodox medicine.

PART ONE

A Natural Alternative

Alternative or complementary medicine offers a very different approach to health care from conventional Western medicine. It is based on the principle that body and mind work as one, and that the whole person must be treated, not just the symptoms or the illness. Before ill-health can be cured, its cause must be found and dealt with. Only when every aspect of a person's life is considered, can a true diagnosis be made and the appropriate treatment prescribed.

Most health problems today are not caused by disease, but by the detrimental effects of our modern diet and lifestyle. Pollution, stress, lack of exercise, caffeine, nicotine, alcohol and a diet high in sugar, fat and highly processed foods are all factors that weaken our constitution and lead to ill-health.

As health-awareness has grown in recent years, so the importance of a balanced diet and a healthy lifestyle has been realised. This has led to a growing interest in alternative therapies, which offer new approaches to diagnosis and treatment and acknowledge the connection between mind and body

Alternative health care encompasses different disciplines, therapies and diagnostic techniques, many of which are interlinked or work together. For easier understanding, it can be grouped into four main categories:

 Complete healing systems like homoeopathy, naturopathy and traditional Chinese medicine

 Diagnostic techniques such as kinesiology and iridology

 Complementary therapies like massage, reflexology and hydrotherapy

 Self-help treatments like yoga, meditation and visualisation

Alternative therapies have not been subjected to same critical scrutiny as orthodox forms of treatment. They are intended to complement not replace conventional health care. We will always need the life-saving drugs and surgery of modern medicine.

With medical resources stretched to the limit, alternative therapies give us time to explore our lives holistically and take responsibility for our own health and wellbeing. When combined with the skills of conventional medicine, we have the best possible health care.

Therapies and Treatments

Acupressure

An ancient massage skill originating from China. Gentle finger pressure is exerted on the meridian points of the body (the channels of magnetic energy connecting major body organs) to stimulate energy flow and the release of endorphins, the body's own pain-killers.

Acupressure helps to relieve a wide range of health problems, including certain allergies, asthma, arthritis, back pain, circulation disorders, depression, digestive problems, insomnia, migraine, nausea and stress. In a recent clinical trial, expectant mums reported a reduced incidence of morning sickness when wearing special acupressure wrist bands, designed to reduce nausea and travel sickness.

Acupuncture

Acupuncture is one of the elements of Chinese medicine and is based on the concept of the body having an invisible energy flow (chi). The energy runs throughout the body along special channels called meridians, which are linked to the internal organs. Pain and illness are believed to be the result of a blockage in the energy flow.

The first consultation may last as long as an hour, as the therapist takes a detailed history of the patient.

Age, lifestyle and diet as well as any symptoms are all carefully considered before any treatment is given.

During a treatment, fine needles are painlessly inserted into acupuncture points along certain body meridians, to unblock, increase or decrease the flow of energy. An improvement usually starts to be felt after about four to six treatments, and sessions may have a relaxing or invigorating effect. Some therapists use electro or laser treatments instead of needles.

Acupuncture is widely recognised as an effective treatment for a broad range of acute and chronic health conditions.

Alexander Technique

A method of health restoration through better posture claiming to enhance the state of mind and body. Bad posture habits are 'unlearned' with the help of qualified practitioners who demonstrate correct ways to sit, stand and walk.

The Alexander Technique has helped many people overcome medical problems including chronic back pain, stress, depression, ulcers, headaches, arthritis and irritable bowel syndrome.

Aromatherapy

A pressure point massage using essential plant oils with therapeutic properties, specifically chosen for each individual after an initial consultation. The oil's unique properties are absorbed through the skin and affect the nervous and circulatory systems of the body.

Aromatherapy massage is a pleasantly therapeutic treatment and particularly effective in relieving stress and tension. Essential oils are potent substances and may be harmful if used undiluted. Some are unsuitable for use in pregnancy.

Art Therapy

A creative therapy that allows participants to work through feelings, thoughts and emotions. When art is used therapeutically, it becomes an acceptable way of releasing inner tensions. Art therapy also increases self-confidence and improves relaxation and concentration. It requires no special artistic talent or skill, just a willingness to express oneself in clay, paints, crayons or oils.

Art therapy is frequently used in the treatment of stress, depression and emotional conditions causing physical side-effects. By exploring emotional problems, stress-related conditions – insomnia, digestive disorders, and headaches – start to improve.

Autogenic Training

A form of relaxation therapy based on a series of six simple mental exercises and carried out in a sitting or reclining position, under the guidance of an autogenic trainer. A relaxed state near hypnosis may be achieved by focusing on different areas of the body.

Exercise 1	Focuses thoughts on the weight of the arms, legs, neck and shoulders
Exercise 2	Concentrates on a feeling of warmth in the limbs
Exercise 3	Concentrates on the heartbeat
Exercise 4	Focuses on breathing awareness
Exercise 5	Focuses on a feeling of warmth in the abdomen
Exercise 6	Concentrates on the coolness of the forehead

From the initial relaxed state, the patient can go on to experience autogenic meditation, which allows deeper access to the subconscious, either with or without the help of the trainer. Autogenic training can be taken to even greater lengths with *modification* (specific problem areas of the body are addressed and instructed to heal themselves), and *neutralisation* (an analytical process to uncover deeper problems).

Autogenic training is useful for treating a wide range of emotional and stress-related conditions.

Ayurvedic Medicine

An ancient Indian system of medicine covering all aspects of physical, mental and emotional health. Ayurvedic philosophy is to prevent disease and maintain health holistically. Three life forces are believed to control all physical and mental processes and must be in balance. These are *kapha* (moon force), *pitta* (sun force) and *vata* (wind force). The system of healing defines seven constitutional types, each requiring its own plan and guidelines for health maintenance. Establishing these individually may be quite complicated.

Prescribed ayurvedic treatments may be *dietary* (specific food regimes) *medicinal* (vegetable and herbal drugs) or *practical* (massage, meditation, yoga, steam baths) and serve four categories of ailment – *accidental*, *mental*, *natural* and *internal physical*. To benefit from this ancient system of medicine, followers must be dedicated, motivated and willing to learn.

Bach Flower Remedies

The invention of Dr Edward Bach, an orthodox doctor and homoeopath. Dr Bach devised 38 flower and plant remedies, each one being a complete system of healing, to treat various emotional states. Safe, effective and completely natural, each remedy is taken as a few drops on the tongue or in water. *Rescue Remedy* is a unique combination of five flower remedies and is used by countless people in times of shock, severe stress and emotional upheaval.

Bach Flower Remedies are sold in 10ml dropper bottles at health food stores and pharmacies. *Rescue Remedy* is available in a larger size and as a cream.

Balneotherapy

The effective and enjoyable use of spa water (usually heated) for treatments and bathing. Balneotherapy is especially good for people suffering from mobility problems, like the elderly, and those recovering from accidents and surgery. Spa water contains different minerals and properties, which are believed to be absorbed through the skin, benefiting various health conditions.

Currently the only therapeutic spa facility in the UK is at Droitwich where the unique brine baths are used for physiotherapy treatments and recreation. Work is being carried out to restore the therapeutic spa at Bath, probably in time for the year 2000.

Therapeutic spas are also found in Europe, Japan, the USA, New Zealand and many other countries of the world.

Bates Eye Method

Bates Method is a natural and non-invasive way to reduce eyestrain and improve sight. It consists of a series of simple eye exercises which are taught by trained Bates Method practitioners, using relaxation, memory, imagination and perception to improve feedback between the eyes and the brain. As the eyes start to function normally, eyestrain is relieved and vision improves.

Biochemics

Biochemics was developed in the 1870s by German homoeopathic physician, Dr William Schuessler, who identified 12 natural mineral (tissue) salts in the body. These are vital to health and must always be correctly balanced.

Although the 12 tissue salts are also listed in the homoeopathic range of medicines and prepared by the same method, biochemics and homoeopathy are actually quite different. Biochemics aims to redress the mineral deficiency believed to be the cause of illness. Homoeopathy follows the 'like cures like' principle, prescribing remedies which would induce the symptoms in a healthy person, taking into account the patient's mental and emotional state.

Biochemic tissue salts can be taken singly to help alleviate various everyday aches and pains, or in a range of 18 combinations, such as *Combination C* for acidity and heartburn, *Combination P* for aching feet and legs and chilblains. The salts are gentle, non-toxic and non habit-forming, but the tablets are lactose-based and should be avoided by anyone with a milk or sugar intolerance.

Biofeedback

Biofeedback is a type of technically-assisted relaxation therapy. Therapists start by teaching relaxation techniques, then use biofeedback machines to let their patients observe the changes in their mental and physical condition (body temperature, heart rate, brain-wave patterns, and so on). Patients are taught ways to assess and control these changes, using visualisation, relaxation, meditation and breathing.

Biofeedback machines merely provide information – they do not affect the body in any way. As the patient learns to recognise and alter his own bodily responses, he is able to avoid conditions like high blood pressure, migraine and anxiety.

Biofeedback training techniques are designed to affect the part of the nervous system controlling digestion, blood pressure, muscular tension and skin temperature, which until recently, were assumed to be involuntary responses.

Biomagnetic Therapy

A system of treatment that combines the principles of acupuncture and osteopathy with the use of magnets. No needles or manipulation are used. Practitioners place small magnets over the main meridians of the body to rebalance equilibrium and energy flow.

Chiropractic

Chiropractic is a profession specialising in the diagnosis, treatment and management of conditions caused by mechanical dysfunction of the joints and their effects on the nervous system.

The manipulative treatment offers effective relief for disorders of the joints, muscles and spinal column. Chiropractic is based on the principle that when bones are misaligned, muscles are strained or even go into spasm and prevent the body from functioning correctly. This affects all the systems of the body, and may cause illness and discomfort.

After taking a full medical history, the chiropractor may take X-rays to confirm the diagnosis. Gentle manipulation is then applied to ease out areas of muscle spasm, pain and tenderness. When normal alignment is restored, the body heals itself.

Chiropractic is one of the most reputable and popular alternative therapies, and increasing numbers of family doctors now refer patients with back problems to chiropractors.

Clinical Ecology

A therapy which helps overcome serious problems of allergies and intolerances to food and other substances. Various techniques are employed to identify sensitivity to food or chemicals. When the culprit food or substance is found appropriate treatment can be advised. Many allergies are difficult to diagnose and some testing techniques are expensive.

Most GPs refer patients with food sensitivities to medically qualified practitioners with a special interest and training in this type of problem.

Clinical Nutrition
(also known as Dietary Therapy)

Clinical nutrition uses diet therapeutically to treat and prevent illness and restore the body to full health and optimum function. Many health problems are triggered by allergies or intolerances to certain foods or by a vitamin or mineral deficiency. Certain foods improve digestion, raise energy levels and decrease mucus production. Changing to a healthier diet can notably improve conditions such as rheumatism, arthritis, asthma and eczema.

Although it should be possible to obtain all the nutrients we need for health from a well-planned diet, pesticides, food processing, storage, cooking and the body's own digestive shortcomings may deplete nutrient levels, causing less than optimum health.

The clinical nutritionist takes a full medical history, paying particular attention to the patient's diet and lifestyle. Hair may be analysed and tests carried out on urine, blood and sweat. Based on the information gathered, a personal diet plan and supplements regime is worked out. Advice may also be given if other treatments are needed to restore health

Clinical nutritionists are often medical doctors with specialist training in nutrition. Non-medical practitioners should have a recognised qualification in nutrition and be registered with a professional society.

Many health problems are solved through clinical nutrition, and the whole body benefits from a healthier more balanced diet. Many naturopaths, homoeopaths and medical herbalists also use dietary therapy as part of their treatment.

Colonic Irrigation

A method of cleansing the lower bowel using purified water to gently flush away accumulated faecal matter, toxic waste, gas and mucus deposits. Once considered a rather bizarre treatment, the benefits of colonic irrigation have achieved a higher profile in recent years, after it become known that the late Princess Diana had regular treatment sessions.

Colour Therapy

Colour therapy is based on the belief that colour has therapeutic properties that affect people in many ways, physically and mentally. Colour affects mood, perception of temperature and time and the ability to concentrate. Colour therapists believe that different colours affect and revitalise certain parts of the body, and that each of the seven colours of the prism – red, orange, yellow, green, blue, indigo and violet – has its own special influence on health. An unhealthy body emits an unbalanced pattern of vibrations, and some illnesses can be helped by changing colour input to the body and restoring balance. Colour is used through light, food and the environment to stimulate production of hormones which control the body's chemical and energy balance.

After the therapist has assessed the colours to be used for treatment of a particular ailment, an instrument beams coloured lights onto the patient, using a main and complementary colour in an irregular rhythm. The therapist may suggest colours to wear and to use in the home and how to visualise treatment colours.

Counselling
(see also Psychotherapy)

Everyone needs to talk over life's problems with a sympathetic and attentive listener. Many difficulties can be eased or even solved by such discussions. Persistent or overwhelming problems may require professional counselling which can be arranged privately or through health practices, churches, Citizens Advice Bureaux or organisations like Relate. Counselling can help with sexual and marital problems, bereavement and most of life's crises.

Counsellors are trained to help their clients come to terms with their problems and take responsibility for themselves. By making changes in their reactions and behaviour, improvements can be made in relationships and life situations.

Cranial Massage/Osteopathy

This alternative treatment involves delicate manipulation of the eight bones of the skull and the facial bones into their correct positions. Even slight bone displacement can cause or contribute to conditions like tinnitus, neuralgia and headaches.

The massage must be carried out by a qualified osteopath who is preferably a medical doctor. Cranial osteopathy has been found helpful in the treatment of migraines, whiplash, head injuries and pain caused by dental work.

Craniosacral Therapy

A bodywork treatment that uses gentle manipulative techniques and palpation to encourage the body to rebalance and heal itself.

Crystal Therapy

Crystals have been treasured throughout history, with ancient civilisations using them to heal and protect. Crystal therapists believe that every crystal has its own unique energies which can be used for healing purposes. Anyone with an open attitude can benefit from crystals, but smokers, alcohol and drug users will be less sensitive to crystalline energies.

Those who feel their lives need direction may find contact with their birthstone helps them become more focused.

Different types of crystals are used for healing physical, emotional and spiritual problems. They can be placed on parts of the body needing treatment or on the pressure points. The positive energy of the semi-precious stones is believed to exert a healing influence.

Dance Movement Therapy

A relatively new therapy for treating psychological and emotional problems through dance movements. The therapy uses the connection between body movement and emotion to express and manage feelings often too deep to express in words.

Therapy sessions may be individual or in groups, with the therapist suggesting movements initially, then encouraging patients to contribute their own ideas. A theme usually emerges from the movements which is explored in greater depth later, when problems are identified and resolved. Music is sometimes used during sessions.

Dowsing

Dowsing is used to diagnose illness or the presence of undesirable additives in food. A bead or object is attached to a thread to create a pendulum and held over the person or food. The theory is that all substances emit 'good' and 'bad' radiation waves which we can quickly learn to identify. The direction in which the pendulum swings in response to questions asked is interpreted as a 'yes' or a 'no' answer. This assists in diagnosing a health problem or identifying a troublesome food.

Electrotherapy

Used mainly in physiotherapy treatments to treat back pain and sports injuries and in some maternity units to relieve pain in childbirth. The mild electrical stimulation activates nerves that block out pain. TENS is the best known form of transcutaneous nerve stimulation, in which a small battery-powered machine sends weak electrical impulses through the skin by means of rubber pads, coated and taped around the area to be treated. TENS machines can be borrowed from hospital physiotherapy departments for outpatient use.

Electro-acupuncture is a form of electrotherapy treatment which uses a machine to pass electrical impulses from up to eight needles into the body. These must be operated by a qualified acupuncturist.

Space technology has led to the development of *Medicur*, another electro-magnetic device for the treatment of pain. This small portable device emits specific magnetic waves, triggering production of endorphins, the body's own pain-killers. These stimulate the nervous system and encourage the body to heal itself. Trials in several UK hospitals have so far yielded dramatic relief from pain caused by arthritis, rheumatism, backache, circulatory disorders and osteoporosis. The device can be used at home and provides natural, safe pain relief.

Fasting

Abstinence from solid food (but not water or fluids) for a certain period of time is best undertaken with professional help. A naturopath may recommend fasting for one or two days a week to cure a specific health problem, or prescribe a longer fast at a health farm or residential clinic.

Unpleasant symptoms like headaches, nausea, bad breath and hunger pangs may occur during the first few days of extended fasts, but are transient. These symptoms are probably an indication that the body is ridding itself of toxins.

When undergoing a fast, patients are advised to take plenty of rest and refrain from energetic exercise.

The Feldenkrais Method

The Feldenkrais Method aims to make movement more useful and efficient by developing new patterns in the brain. It uses gentle and interesting movement sequences to stimulate the exploratory learning of our formative years. This enables improvements to be made in the quality of everyday movements. The Feldenkrais Method uses two specific techniques: *Awareness Through Movement*, taught in classes to make participants conscious of their own patterns and new possibilities; and *Functional Integration*, which uses gentle manipulation to do the same, on a one-to-one basis.

The Feldenkrais Method (named after its inventor, Dr Mosche Feldenkrais) claims to enhance life and improve wellbeing whatever your age, ability or state of health.

Classes last between 45 minutes and an hour and help posture, breathing and circulation. They are especially useful to nurses, athletes, dancers, musicians and anyone whose lifestyle involves a lot of specific movement.

Food Combining – the Hay Diet

William Hay, an American doctor, devised this unique diet to combat digestive problems. It is based on the principle that carbohydrates (starches and sugars) should not be eaten at the same time as proteins and acid fruits. The theory is that protein stimulates the production of acid in the stomach, and may interfere with carbohydrate digestion which requires an alkaline medium. Food is categorised into three groups: proteins, carbohydrates and neutral foods, which may be eaten with either of the other two groups.

Adjusting to the Hay diet may seem odd at first (no food combinations such as fish and chips, meat and potatoes or biscuits and cheese). When trying the diet for the first time, it helps to have a categorised list of basic foods and some menu suggestions. These can be found in several books now available on the subject. Many people have benefited from a food combining regime, which not only relieves digestive symptoms but also eases some types of arthritic joint pains. As a further bonus, excess weight tends to be shed without recourse to dieting.

Healing

This is a general term for a therapy that uses touch as a means of transferring healing energy from healer to patient. The healer is the channel for the transfer of this energy which can also be effected by meditation. Some healers believe their powers of healing come from an outside 'spiritual' source. When this feeling is shared with the patient, the cure may be quicker and more effective.

Health Resorts

Modern health resorts offer relaxation in pleasant surroundings and the chance to reassess health and lifestyle. The food is generally of a high standard, tasty and fresh, yet low in fat and calories. Famous for their laid-back ambience and pampering treatments, health resorts also offer extensive fitness facilities. A daily timetable offers exercise classes for every age and ability as well as supervised gyms, swimming pools, tennis courts, bicycles, escorted walks and even country hikes.

On arrival, visitors have a consultation with a nurse or therapist to discuss the aims of the visit, and then a

The Really Useful Guide to Natural Health and Beauty

schedule of treatments and activities is drawn up. Although health resorts tend to be expensive, the daily rate usually includes a number of treatments, all meals, accommodation and full use of the facilities. A short stay at a health resort is great way to unwind and may even provide the incentive needed to start living a healthier more active lifestyle.

Herbal Medicine

The medicinal use of herbs is as old as mankind itself and herbal medicine is the oldest system of healing, originating in China more than five thousand years ago. Even today, herbalism is three to four times more commonly practised throughout the world than conventional medicine, and more than 15 percent of all medical prescriptions are plant-based.

Like all forms of alternative healthcare, herbalism treats the patient holistically. The first session lasts about an hour, and includes taking a detailed health and lifestyle history from the patient. Prescribed herbal treatments are always tailored to individual need, taking into account all aspects of a patient's life.

Herbalism is especially effective when used to complement conventional medical treatment and to improve chronic health conditions such as arthritis, asthma, rheumatism, digestive disorders, high blood pressure, migraine, neuralgia, varicose veins, viral infections and skin problems.

Homoeopathy

A medically recognised and popular complete system of alternative medicine, based on the principle that 'like cures like'. Homoeopathic treatment is very complex, as every aspect of the patient's diet, lifestyle and personality is taken into consideration as well as the symptoms or illness.

After making a diagnosis, the homoeopath chooses a remedy for the individual symptoms. By prescribing minute amounts of substances known to cause similar symptoms to the those of the patient, the body is stimulated to heal itself. These tiny doses prevent the symptoms becoming worse (as larger doses would) and are prepared from highly diluted and special forms of plant, mineral and animal substances. Homoeopathic remedies are so dilute they can be taken safely by everyone and have no side-effects. Unusually, in homoeopathy, the more dilute the dosage, the more effective the cure. Symptoms may temporarily become worse after taking homoeopathic remedies. This is interpreted as a good sign and indicate that the body is starting the healing process.

Homoeopathy can be used by everyone for most medical conditions. However, conventional treatment should always be sought first for any health problem.

Hydrotherapy

Therapeutic treatment involving the external use of water in its application. Hydrotherapy includes many different forms of treatment: bathing or exercising muscles and joints in a warm therapeutic pool; hot and cold compresses to reduce swelling and inflammation and to improve blood flow to diseased areas; warm water immersion; cold water wraps for various disorders; hot and cold baths; jet sprays and inhalation therapy to aid respiratory problems.

Heated thermal baths are sadly neglected in Britain but used extensively in European spas, along with modified exercise routines to aid arthritis and mobility. Bathing in warm spa water cleanses the pores, improves circulation and exercises the muscles.

Immersion in water has profound physiological effects, caused by the volume of blood pooled in the calves being returned to the heart. Research indicates that hydrotherapy sessions may be an effective way of avoiding the common cold.

To get maximum benefit from hydrotherapy, bathers should relax for about 30 minutes after a pool session and take care getting out of the water. Immersion in hot/warm water lowers blood pressure and may cause dizziness.

Hypnotherapy

Hypnotherapy is believed to work by tapping into the trance-like state between wakefulness and deep sleep. Exactly how this happens is still not fully understood, but obviously the mind controls the functions and health of the body.

During the initial consultation which is likely to last about an hour, the hypnotherapist enquires about all aspects of the patient's lifestyle, including eating habits and health problems. After discussing the aims of the treatment, the patient is encouraged to relax in a comfortable position then, through repeated instructions, is brought to an even deeper state of relaxation. The subconscious mind can then focus on the problem in hand and take in suggestions from the hypnotherapist to change inappropriate thoughts, behaviour and feelings. In this state of profound relaxation, painful treatments and dental procedures can be carried out without any pain being felt by the patient.

Although its use as a television entertainment may have tarnished its image, there can be little doubt that hypnotherapy helps many people. It helps cure bad habits and behavioural difficulties like smoking, drug misuse, eating disorders, compulsions and phobias.

Hypnotherapy is also used to treat childbirth pain, skin disorders, migraine, IBS, and other conditions caused by anxiety and stress

Hypnotherapy is a useful tool in the hands of a reputable therapist, with whom the patient feels comfortable and confident.

Ionisation

Air becomes ionised – electrically charged – as a result of certain environmental factors like pollution, electrical appliances, air conditioning or even dust. While negative ions are invigorating – formed in nature by fresh air, running water and lightning – a surplus of positive ions creates a heavy and tense atmosphere, as happens before a storm.

City air contains very few negatively charged ions. Asthma sufferers and those with chest and lung problems, who are sensitive to poor quality air, may find an ioniser helpful. These small electrical devices use little energy to produce a constant stream of refreshing negative ions and can be safely left on all night. They are available from health food and department stores and larger pharmacies.

Iridology

A non-invasive diagnostic technique that interprets the markings on the irises of the eye to highlight potential health problems. The iris (the coloured part of the eye) is believed to mirror the body's state of health, being the recipient of messages from thousands of tiny nerve endings from all over the body. These register on the iris, allowing levels of toxicity and inflammation to be seen when the eye's colour, fibres and structure are studied. The iris records only the state of the various organs and tissues, not specific diseases. The right eye reflects the right-hand side of the body, the left eye the left-hand side.

The iris is examined with a torch and magnifying glass and may be photographed. The markings are then explained and discussed with the patient. Depending on what the examination reveals, the iridologist may offer dietary and lifestyle advice or suggest that the patients sees their own doctor.

👁 Kinesiology

Applied kinesiology uses gentle muscle testing to discover and cure energy blockages and imbalances in all parts of the body. Restoring balance to the energy channels stimulates the body's natural healing processes. Practitioners use light touch to diagnose blocked energy, and may give a shiatsu or acupressure massage to release it and correct imbalances in the body. Dietary advice may also be given at the end of the session.

Kinesiology is widely used to monitor the effects of foods on the body and to identify allergies.

👁 Kirlian Photography

Named after its Russian inventors, this form of high voltage photography claims to produce prints of a person's electromagnetic field (aura), revealing their mental and physical state. The aura's colour and brightness is interpreted by the practitioner to diagnose weaknesses and illness before symptoms appear.

❋ Macrobiotics

The macrobiotic way of life originated in Japan and is based on the Chinese yin-yang principle. It balances a diet based on wholegrain cereals and vegetables (no white rice, flour or refined sugar products) with exercise and environmental awareness. A macrobiotic diet, although restricted, is very health-giving and may be undertaken to prevent or treat serious illnesses like cancer.

Much emphasis is placed on correct cooking utensils, ideally cast iron pots and pans that distribute the heat evenly. Copper and aluminium utensils are unsuitable for macrobiotic cooking, as traces of these metals may affect the food's vitamin content.

Magnetic Therapy
(see also Biomagnetic Therapy and Electrotherapy)

The application of a magnetic force on the body to treat chronic and acute health problems. Practitioners claim the use of magnets increases the supply of oxygen and nutrients to the cells and speeds up the healing process.

Manual Lymphatic Drainage
(MLD)

A unique massage treatment which uses subtle techniques to stimulate the lymphatic system, part of the body's immune system. The therapist uses light circular movements on the patient to encourage the flow of lymph and help disperse waste fluids and toxins that have accumulated in the tissues.

Treatment sessions last about an hour and several sessions may be required to improve chronic conditions like sinusitis and lymphoedema or to promote the healing of fractures and wounds.

Massage

A popular 'hands on' treatment to improve and maintain the balance and health of all body systems. Massage promotes relaxation and is an effective treatment for stress-related tension. It can also be used to treat problems associated with the muscular/skeletal system.

Although most types of body massage require undressing (to underpants at least), the patient's modesty is always respected. Towels are draped over the patient and only the part of the body being treated is exposed at any one time.

Certain massage therapies aim to improve health problems and encourage the body to heal itself. These include aromatherapy, Rolfing, sports massage, Hellerwork, lymphatic drainage massage and various types of oriental massage techniques.

Meditation *(see also Yoga)*

Meditation uses the power of concentration to calm and slow down the body and to control thoughts. It can be practised in a group or alone and is easily learned.

Allow about ten to 20 minutes daily for the purpose. Choose a quiet room where you are not likely to be disturbed and disconnect the telephone. Sit comfortably upright with the eyes open and hands resting in your lap. Consciously rid your mind of stimulating thoughts or worries, and think instead of a single pleasing image. Try to ignore any intruding thoughts. The mind can be focused on breathing, relaxing or even on a favourite photograph or object. Playing a soothing meditation tape will help create the right frame of mind for relaxation.

Megavitamin Therapy

The basis of megavitamin therapy is the supervised consumption of large amounts of vitamins to prevent or cure certain illnesses. American biochemist Linus Pauling first attracted attention to this theory when his studies claimed that large doses of vitamin C could ward off the common cold. His research into other vitamins and minerals led him to name this new approach to health *Orthomolecular Medicine*. This work was based on maintaining or restoring good health by establishing each individual's correct levels of vitamins and minerals.

Other American doctors had previously used large doses of vitamin B3 successfully to treat patients with schizophrenia. This led to a whole new area of orthomolecular psychiatry being developed to treat mental illness.

Megavitamin therapy is now the usual term for this type of treatment for physical and mental problems. It must always be supervised, as overdosing on any nutrient may be dangerous. Practitioners of the therapy believe that anyone suffering from an illness is likely to have metabolic abnormalities caused by a lack of vitamins, and will therefore benefit from the treatment. The therapy is also helpful for those who suffer from poor absorption of nutrients, suffer from certain illnesses, or are undergoing medical treatment that increases vitamin need .

Metamorphic Technique

This is a unique type of communication through gentle manipulation of the feet, hands and head. The technique is based on the relationship between the foot and the nine months of gestation. Practitioners use circular finger movements to manipulate the inner side of the foot, the ankle and big toe. The outside edge of the thumb down to the wrist is massaged, as well as the bony ridges on the head. The technique claims to help those who feel their lives are blocked in some way or who have a recurring health problem. Children and those born with a handicap derive particular benefit from metamorphic technique.

Naturopathy

Naturopathy is a complete health care system, offering a natural approach through its philosophy, lifestyle and health programmes. Naturopathy is based on the belief that the body has the ability to heal itself when harmful toxins are eliminated. Poor eating habits and an unhealthy lifestyle cause toxins to accumulate. Naturopaths use only natural cures like massage, exercise, therapeutic diets, hydrotherapy and supervised fasting, to stimulate the body's natural defences and restore balance and health.

Naturopathy is especially effective for the treatment of chronic disorders and digestive problems caused by a poor diet. The naturopathic diet is based on simple wholefoods, fruit and vegetables and helps to detoxify the body. Meat is excluded, as are all processed, highly refined and artificially sweetened foods and stimulants like tea and coffee.

Many people experience increased energy levels, greater physical fitness and improved immunity to infection, by changing to a more naturopathic lifestyle.

Neuro Linguistic Programming
(NLP)

A technique that has deservedly become popular because it improves communications on both personal and business levels. It builds confidence and allows a person more control and influence over his/her life.

NLP is easy to learn and its positive approach ensures quick results for certain types of problem. It is particularly effective when used to overcome phobias and old fears that prevent life being enjoyed to the full. NLP opens up new ways of thinking and reacting to life's situations, with new possibilities and choices.

Nutritional Therapy

A useful therapy offering individual diet advice and supplement regimes to correct nutritional deficiencies and combat allergies. Nutritional therapy helps reduce the number of toxins in the body, enhancing health and wellbeing.

Osteopathy

One of the most widely accepted 'alternative' practices. Like chiropractic, osteopathy works on the physical structure of the body, using manipulation, massage and stretching techniques to overcome a variety of conditions and illnesses. It is well-known for its successful treatment of back pain, and certain techniques that cause loud clicks and pops of the vertebrae and joints!

Some osteopaths also practise cranial osteopathy, which involves gently manipulating the hairline joints of the skull bones. The technique corrects any slight misalignment which may be causing symptoms such as tinnitus, headaches and migraine.

After taking a detailed health history, the patient removes any tight clothing and lies down for an examination. The osteopath may also take X-rays to aid the diagnosis. Some conditions require only a single treatment to relieve painful symptoms, while others need several sessions. Osteopathy improves circulation to all parts of the body and is often more effective at treating back pain than orthodox medicine.

Pilates

An exercise and movement method designed to improve posture and increase muscular strength and suppleness. Pilates exercise involves one-to-one training using the body's own weight resistance against gravity and pulleys. This strengthens weaker muscles groups and lengthens bulkier ones. The movements are slow, repetitive and very controlled. Pilates is popular with dancers and athletes as it can be used to gradually change the shape of the body.

Polarity Therapy

Polarity therapy incorporates various Eastern and Western healing techniques and counselling. Like traditional Chinese medicine, polarity therapy is based on the subtle balance of yin and yang and the interaction of opposites. It also shares the same philosophy as other oriental therapies, believing that optimum health is only enjoyed when the body is in balance and the vital energy force flows unimpeded throughout the body's meridians. Imbalances, energy blockages and stagnation are believed to be the sole cause of illness and disease.

Polarity therapy requires changes in the patient's diet, exercise and attitudes to health and healing. The first session includes a lengthy consultation when all aspects of the patient's health and lifestyle are discussed. Treatments are aimed at stimulating the body's powers of self-healing.and include fasting and cleansing diets, manipulation, therapeutic touch, stretching postures and counselling.

Psychotherapy
(see also Counselling)

Psychotherapy is an umbrella term covering many different talking therapies, including cognitive, eclectic and Gestault therapy, NLP, transactional analysis and hypnotherapy. As in counselling, the client is encouraged to talk about and come to terms with their problems, guided by the therapist. The client is helped to examine the root cause of their difficulties in greater depth than in counselling.

Psychotherapy's aim is self-discovery – finding the origins of problems and negative behaviour patterns and helping the client build on their own character strengths.

Many health problems result from emotional difficulties, so working through these often brings about an improvement in physical health.

When choosing a trained therapist, it is important to find someone with whom you feel comfortable and at ease. You must be able to trust them sufficiently to disclose your innermost feelings and worries.

Psychology's many benefits include an increased sense of wellbeing, greater self-knowledge and confidence.

Radionics

A means of diagnosing a person's health indirectly. Like many other alternative therapies, radionics is based on the need to have an unimpeded flow of energy through the invisible channels or meridians of the body. Radionics believes that every person has a unique energy pattern and rhythm. All body cells reflect these vibrations, which change when the energy flow is blocked or there is ill health. This altered pattern can be read from any part of the body and is treated by sending coded messages using a special machine or a pendulum.

The patient supplies a personal item, like a lock of hair or a nail clipping, and completes a detailed health questionnaire. After studying this, the practitioner puts the items in a box with dials and magnets to pick up energy vibrations, or he may swing a pendulum over the personal items and a diagram or chart of the body. When the practitioner feels a resistance on the dials, or the pendulum reacts, he/she can ascertain the health of the different body organs or particular problem areas highlighted in the questionnaire. Coded messages are then sent back to the patient, through the box, correcting any imbalances detected by the energy vibrations.

Although radionics has its followers, it is one of the least understood alternative therapies.

Reflexology
(see also Zone Therapy)

Reflexology is based on the principle that the body's anatomy is reflected in miniature on the feet and hands. This popular treatment involves massaging and applying pressure to certain points on the hands and feet, which correspond to the different organs of the body.

The body is divided into ten energy zones, each passing through the body from the top of the head to the tips of the fingers and toes, with five zones on the left and five on the right. Each organ, structure and gland is represented along one or more of these zones at reflex points which correspond to the anatomy of the body.

A therapist works by treating the whole foot or hand, specialising on the reflex points that show a reaction. Every treatment is tailored to suit the individual needs of the patient. By applying special foot massage techniques, almost any organ or body area can be treated.

Reflexology helps many common ailments, including back pain, sinus problems, migraine, stress and digestive problems. It should not be used to treat undiagnosed acute pain or fever.

Reiki

A Japanese system of healing and meditation, used to help various mental and physical conditions brought about by emotional upsets, a poor diet or stress. The therapy has five principles:

> *Just for today do not worry*
> *Just for today do not anger*
> *Honour your parents, teachers and elders*
> *Earn your living honestly*
> *Show gratitude to every living thing*

In Reiki, the practitioner becomes a channel for the transfer of healing energy into the recipient. No belief in theory or dogma is necessary for the therapy to work – all that is required is for the patient to want to be healed. Reiki is believed to help all forms of illness by boosting energy at every level: mental, physical, emotional and spiritual.

During a treatment, the patient relaxes, fully clothed, on a couch or bed. The practitioner gently places his or her hands in a sequence of positions covering the patient's whole body. As energy flows out of the practitioner's hands and into the patient, the recipient's own energy stimulates a healing response. This may cause a pleasant feeling of warmth, tingling and relaxation.

Relaxation Techniques

Regular periods of relaxation are essential for physical and mental health. Some relaxation techniques require special training, others can be self-taught, like deep breathing, tensing and relaxing the muscles and clearing the mind. Relaxation is often practised at the end of an energetic exercise session, prolonging and enhancing the beneficial effects of exercising. Yoga, massage, aromatherapy and meditation are all forms of relaxation.

Shiatsu

A Japanese massage technique similar to acupressure and based on the same principles and traditions as other Eastern therapies.

The patient dresses in loose clothing and lies on a large mat on the floor. The practitioner gives the massage by pressing along the meridian lines of the body using his/her elbows, knees, feet, palms and fingers. Shiatsu restores balance and 'oneness' by summoning energy to and from parts of the body that need it. Highly effective in the relief of insomnia, pain and tension.

Spa treatments
(see Balneotherapy)

Use of spas (therapeutic mineral springs) declined in Britain with the founding of the National Health Service and the growth of the pharmaceutical industry. The British Spas Federation was formed to develop wider public understanding and interest in the benefits of spa-related tourism and culture. Currently the brine water spa at Droitwich is the only therapeutic spa operating in the UK. Bath's spa is due to reopen shortly with updated treatment facilities.

Around the world, spas continue to prosper, providing therapeutic medical treatments with first class recreational facilities in attractive locations. Spa travel consultants can arrange visits to overseas therapeutic spas suited to particular health needs.

T'ai-chi Ch'un
(usually called T'ai-chi)

Originating in Chinese culture, but now practised all over the world, T'ai-chi is meditation in motion. Participants perform slow-moving, circular, dance-like movements as they focus on the body and their mental and emotional states. The graceful flowing movements are best carried out in the open air, encouraging relaxation and a feeling of 'letting go'. T'ai-chi also helps improve breathing and posture, tones up the body and stimulates circulation. Classes are now available at evening institutes and leisure centres nationwide.

Traditional Chinese Medicine

Traditional Chinese medicine is relatively new to Britain, although its theories and philosophies have been practised in China for thousands of years.

Traditional Chinese medicine (TCM) is a highly sophisticated and complex healing system which uses a range of therapies in its application, notably acupuncture, massage, diet therapy, exercise and herbalism. It is based on the concept that good health depends on an invisible flow of energy (chi), which provides vitality and fights illness. This energy flows along 14 paths or meridians, each connected to a major organ. The meridians link all parts of the body together and have 365 main pressure points which relate to specific body organs.

The philosophy of TCM is that we are all controlled by opposing but complementary forces known as yin and yang. Seven of the meridian acupuncture points are yin and the remaining seven yang. The body, its organs, the mind and emotions are all subject to the opposing influences of yin (female, passive, dark, negative) and yang (male, active, light, positive). TCM aims to restore an uninterrupted flow of energy, as blockages in the meridians are believed to cause illness and disease and result in an imbalance of yin and yang.

A first consultation involves taking a detailed health history, with questions asked about all aspects of diet and lifestyle. After this, the tongue is examined and a pulse reading taken. All this information enables the practitioner to decide on a course of treatment to restore chi and get the body back in balance.

Some skin conditions like eczema have proved untreatable by conventional medicine, but shown an amazing response to treatment with prescribed Chinese herbs. As some Chinese herbs are extremely toxic, self-medication is not recommended. Chinese herbs should always be prescribed by a qualified practitioner.

Visualisation Therapy

This interesting therapy encourages the patient to use positive imaginative thoughts to benefit health and self-esteem. Easy to learn, it can be used in many different situations to overcome mental and physical problems. Visualisation is based on the belief that mind and body affect each other directly. Thoughts have physical as well as mental effects. Physical sensations and even feelings, can be influenced when their perception is changed.

There is no national register of therapists as visualisation is used in conjunction with other treatments such as hypnotherapy or psychotherapy.

Vitamin Supplements

In theory, people in good health, who eat a sensible diet with plenty of fruit and vegetables should not need to take vitamin or mineral supplements. In reality, the nutritional quality of food is adversely affected by factors like environmental pollution and intensive farming methods that use insecticides and chemicals. Taking a daily multi-vitamin/mineral tablet is a simple safeguard against most deficiencies. Pregnant and menopausal women benefit from extra vitamins and minerals, as well as the elderly, vegans, vegetarians, women taking the contraceptive pill, convalescents and anyone with a stressful lifestyle or eating a poor quality diet. Health food stores, mail order companies and pharmacies can advise suitable brands for individual needs.

Yin and Yang

Most alternative therapies are based on the Chinese concept of yin and yang, the two opposing but complementary forces, which make up the complete whole. Good health requires a person's yin and yang to be in perfect balance.

Practitioners use oriental diagnosis to assess which force is deficient. This involves taking a detailed history of the patient's health, diet and lifestyle and carrying out two particular procedures - a pulse diagnosis and an examination of the tongue.

Yoga

Yoga originated in India and is a system of

spiritual, mental and physical training. There are several different aspects of yoga – the best known in Western countries is the physical Hatha yoga. This includes various postures and exercises that alternatively stretch and release tension in the muscles, enhancing physical and mental wellbeing and relaxation. Learning to breathe correctly is important, as the breath is considered to be a person's *prana* or life force. Yoga teaches control of mind and body – no one is too old to enjoy the benefits of practising it.

Zone Therapy

Zone therapy is now called reflexology. Originally devised by an American surgeon, who divided the body into ten energy channels and then applied healing pressure to certain points on these channels with his hands or special instruments. The zones extended from the toes up through the body to the head and back again, covering each organ and part of the body. As the therapy evolved, practitioners treated the body by concentrating on the feet rather than on the different areas (zones) .

PART TWO

Health Conditions Helped by Complementary Therapies

Acne

The scourge of adolescent years! Caused by hormonal changes and overactivity of the sebaceous glands of the face, neck and back. This results in unsightly spots, lumps, whiteheads and blackheads. Orthodox medical treatment includes vitamin A derivatives, long-term antibiotics and topical applications of powerful gels and lotions. Most cases clear up completely by the early 20s although, in severe cases, the skin may be left permanently pitted and scarred.

Sufferers can help themselves by keeping the skin scrupulously clean. Acne is not generally thought to be related to diet, but cutting down on sugar and animal fats and eating wholemeal bread and fresh fruit and vegetables is more beneficial than a diet of junk and convenience foods. Drinking several glasses of filtered or mineral water every day helps to detoxify the body and clear the skin.

Certain nutritional supplements are known to help acne. These include zinc (30mg daily) which has important skin-healing properties; beta carotene (50,000 to 100,000iu daily); selenium (200mcg daily); and vitamin E (400iu daily). Alternative therapies for acne include Bach Flower Remedies, herbal treatments, homoeopathy and the application of tea tree oil.

Allergy

The body's abnormal creation of antidotes to certain substances (allergens) which it comes into contact with. These allergens (metals, clothing, chemicals and foods) generally have no unpleasant effects on the first encounter, but cause the body to make antibodies. At subsequent encounters, the antibodies react to these culprit allergens by producing the chemical histamine, which causes the symptoms of asthma, eczema, hay fever and skin rashes.

Many health practitioners now recognise that food allergies (also known as food intolerances) are likely to be associated with a wide range of disorders. Allergies to wheat and dairy products are particularly common. Many private and NHS clinics provide help with elimination diets and offer food allergy testing.

Alternative treatments to diagnose and treat allergies include kinesiology, homoeopathy, clinical ecology and ionisation.

Arthritis

Alternative medicine offers many different remedies for this painful affliction, which affects people of all ages but especially those in the middle and later years. There are many different types of arthritis and all involve some disorder or inflammation of the joints.

The most common forms are osteoarthritis, caused by wear and tear on the joints, and rheumatoid arthritis, an illness affecting the body's immune system. Gout is another type of arthritis, caused by crystals of uric acid collecting in the sufferer's joints.

All arthritis sufferers should recognise the importance of eating a healthy balanced diet. Many people find their symptoms are eased by cutting down on acid-forming foods like red meat, white sugar, dairy produce, citrus fruits, salt and coffee.

Painful symptoms may be improved by taking a suitable nutritional supplement. Fish oils, green-lipped mussel extract, evening primrose oil, selenium with vitamins A, C and E and the herbal remedy devil's claw have variously been found effective by sufferers.

Alternative therapies may also alleviate symptoms; homoeopathy, herbal medicine, acupuncture and manipulative therapies like osteopathy, chiropractic and reflexology, have all been used with good results. Physiotherapy and hydrotherapy are excellent treatments for arthritis, as they improve circulation and mobility in painful joints. Regular moderate exercise, especially swimming, is also beneficial. European spas specialise in thermal treatments for arthritis which are medically prescribed and supervised.

Breast Pain

Tender, swollen and painful breasts are experienced by many women before a period. The condition may be relieved by taking evening primrose oil, a rich source of gamma linolenic acid (an essential fatty acid) with many health benefits, or a magnesium supplement. In trials conducted by PREMSOC (the Premenstrual Society), premenstrual breast pain was significantly reduced by magnesium supplementation. Both supplements are available from health food stores and pharmacies. Reducing intakes of caffeine, alcohol, salt and salty foods is also helpful.

Cellulite

Cellulite is the trendy word for the body fat that appears on most women's bodies as they approach the menopause. Cellulite causes the thighs, bottom, upper arms and stomach to appear lumpy and dimpled. It is difficult to shift, but gradual loss of weight while taking regular exercise, switching to a 75 percent raw food diet and drinking plenty of water, may help. Skin-brushing with a natural bristle brush or friction glove before taking a morning bath or shower stimulates the lymphatic system and encourages removal of toxins and cellulite.

Topical cellulite creams are expensive and may even firm up the skin but they cannot get rid of fat. This can only be permanently removed by surgery or liposuction, an expensive and often painful procedure that uses strong suction to force out fat cells. New and less drastic non-invasive treatments are available in beauty salons and health resorts, using ultrasonic techniques to combat cellulite. These promise good results and incorporate personal dietary and lifestyle advice.

Chronic Fatigue Syndrome
(also known as Myalgic Encephalomyelitis [ME] and Post-viral Fatigue)

This mysterious, exhausting illness affects mainly young adults and commonly starts after a virus infection like 'flu or glandular fever. Orthodox medicine offers little in the way of a cure or effective treatment.

Symptoms include acute fatigue, painful muscles, sweating, loss of memory, depression and mood swings. The illness takes anything from a few months to several years to run its course, and may recur.

Certain alternative therapies have been found helpful in treating ME, including:

- **acupuncture**
  treatment aimed at stimulating the immune system;

- **aromatherapy oils for bathing**
  lavender (alleviates tiredness and soothes), *lemon* (promotes refreshing sleep), orange or *geranium* (uplifting and stimulating);

- **Bach Flower Remedies**
  wild rose to combat exhaustion, *crab apple* to purify the system, *clematis* to increase vitality, *heather* to alleviate depressive symptoms;

- **herbal medicines as relaxants and tonics**
  skullcap, wild oats, vervain & *St John's wort;*

- **homoeopathy treatments**
  (individually prescribed);

- **naturopathy**
  recommends radical long-term change to a basic wholefood diet, plenty of rest and fresh air and boosting the immune system with vitamin and mineral supplements.

Cold Sores

Small blisters usually appearing on the lips are caused by the herpes simplex virus. This highly contagious virus may also attack other parts of the face and genitals (genital herpes).

Most adults carry the virus, which is commonly

passed on during childhood and remains dormant in the body, often for years. Fever, stress, exposure to sun or cold can reactivate it at any time.

All pharmacies sell medications to clear up the symptoms of cold sores. Alternative treatments include vitamin supplements and the homoeopathic remedies *Rhus tox.* and *Nat mur.* A new natural preparation for cold sores is also available, based on extracts of the *melissa* herb. Regular use as part of a healthy lip care programme can help prevent cold sores occurring. It is also useful for those who find this painful condition is triggered by sunbathing or exposure to cold temperatures.

Cystitis

Most women have experienced the distressing symptoms of cystitis – the burning pain of passing frequent drops of scalding urine. Cystitis occurs when bacteria from the anus travel up the urinary passage (the urethra) into the bladder and inflame the bladder lining. The condition is less common in men because anal bacteria have further to travel to reach the bladder. Medical advice should be sought for this painful condition as, untreated, cystitis can lead to kidney problems. Most doctors treat cystitis with antibiotic drugs to kill off bladder bacteria.

At the first sign of an attack, sufferers should drink a pint of water or camomile tea to flush out the bladder. The urine can be made less acidic by adding a teaspoon of bicarbonate of soda to a glass of water and drinking the solution every three hours. During an attack, all foods containing acid, vinegar or animal proteins should be avoided, so citrus fruit, eggs, fish, meat and cheese should not be consumed.

Other helpful remedies include home-made barley

water, which has a soothing and diuretic effect, and the homoeopathic remedies *cantharis, staphysagria, aconite* and *sarsaparilla*.

To prevent further attacks, cranberry juice should be taken regularly or cranberry extract tablets. Unique properties in the juice discourage harmful bacteria from sticking to the bladder wall. Anyone prone to cystitis attacks should develop a regular habit of drinking several glasses of water a day.

Depression

The feeling of being 'down in the dumps' is known to all of us, especially when sad or unpleasant events happen that make it hard to cope with life's usual routine. Depression may be experienced after surgery or an illness like 'flu, after childbirth or during the menopause or after some important life event like a bereavement or divorce. We can usually overcome our depressive feelings by talking about them with a sympathetic listenener, or by having something positive to look forward to.

When the depression persists, or if the sufferer seems without hope or talks of suicide, then medical help must be sought immediately. Depression is a serious condition, but usually improves rapidly with treatment. Depressed people often have lowered levels of brain chemicals like serotonin, which affect mood. The new anti-depressant drugs raise these levels, making the sufferer feel better and more likely to benefit from psychotherapy to find the cause of the depression. Depression may be *reactive*, when caused by external factors like grief or redundancy, or *endogenous*, when the cause is internal or unknown.

Depression can be helped by various alternative treatments: Homoeopathic remedies *Arsen.alb.* and

Nat.mur, taken in the 6th potency (6x is the strength usually sold), three times daily; Bach Flower Remedies (*willow, gorse, larch, sweet chestnut* and *walnut*), and aromatherapy massage with specific oils (*basil, neroli, camomile, rose* and *thyme*). The herb *St John's wort* contains an active ingredient hypericin, which has remarkable antidepressant properties. This is now available as a tablet containing standardised hypericin extracts. Large doses of vitamin B6 are sometimes prescribed by alternative practitioners to counteract depression caused by mood changes.

Eczema

A troublesome inflammatory skin condition, common in childhood and causing persistent itchiness with weeping blisters that form dry scabs and crusts. Like asthma, eczema is triggered by an allergic reaction of the body's immune system. Conventional medical treatment includes testing for allergies with skin patches and the application of topical corticosteroid creams to affected areas.

Traditional Chinese medicine has been found to be particularly effective in treating skin conditions like eczema and psoriasis. Acupressure, diet therapy, massage and Chinese herbs may be used to bring the body back into balance and restore the skin's condition.

Hair Loss

The condition of the hair and scalp reflects the body's state of health. Dull, lifeless hair indicates a lack of vitamins and nutrients in the diet which can usually be corrected. However, despite a healthy diet, the hair tends to become thinner with age, and many men experience baldness of the scalp.

There is still no cure for baldness, despite various topical treatments on the market claiming to halt hair loss. Special food and herbal supplements also promise a healthy regrowth of hair over previously bald areas of the scalp plus improved condition of skin and nails. These long-term supplements are expensive, but some people claim to have benefited from them. They are available from pharmacies and health food stores.

Immune System

The complex defence system of the body is made up of special body cells, organs and a network of lymph vessels and capillaries. Our all-important immune system defends the body against invasion by harmful environmental micro-organisms and germs. Without this defence, these would quickly prove fatal.

We can help safeguard and maintain an efficient immune system by eating a nourishing diet and living a healthy lifestyle. During times of stress or illness, the immune system should be boosted with a herbal tonic and a quality antioxidant vitamin/mineral supplement.

Irritable Bowel Syndrome

Irritable bowel syndrome (IBS) is one of modern life's most troublesome complaints. It commonly affects young and middle-aged adults leading busy, stressful lives.

As the muscles of the bowel are controlled by the autonomic nervous system, the condition is caused or made worse by anxiety, stress and nervous disorders. The symptoms – spasmodic pain and bouts of diarrhoea, constipation and wind – are caused by the rapid contractions of the bowel muscles, aggravated by an unbalanced diet and food intolerances.

The alternative approach to treating IBS is to

examine the diet to rule out food sensitivities, and to avoid stimulants like coffee, strong spices and alcohol. Homoeopathic remedies for IBS include *Colocynthis 6* or *30* and *Argentum nit 6* – both remedies to be taken four times a day for two weeks. Hot infusions of peppermint and camomile with a little ginger added are soothing to the irritated bowel. In Europe, oil of peppermint has been used successfully to treat IBS, and capsules and tablets are now widely available in UK health stores. Sufferers should also aim to consume more dietary fibre and attempt to relieve the underlying stress in their lives – yoga exercises are an enjoyable form of relaxation .

Conventional medical treatment for IBS is with antispasmodic drugs which have a calming effect on the bowel muscles. Recent research indicates that some cases are caused by an enzyme deficiency in the digestive tract. This can be tested and corrected with suitable medication.

Joint problems
(see Arthritis)

Most joint problems are caused by some form of arthritis. Joints gradually become less flexible with age, due to natural wear and tear, so good nutrition plays an increasingly vital role in maintaining joint mobility. Extensive research suggests that fish oils containing omega-3 fatty acids may help to ease joint pain and stiffness.

Injuries also inflict damage a limb's tough, fibrous ligaments, causing acute pain, inflammation and weakness. Most joint problems benefit from hydrotherapy – treatments include hot and cold baths, packs, fango, warm paraffin wax, massage and special exercises in a warm pool. Homoeopathy remedies for stiffness and aching limbs include *Rhus. tox, Colchicum* and *Dulcamara*.

Menopause

The time in a woman's life when the ovaries stop producing eggs and fertility declines – a phase that normally occurs between the mid 40s and early 50s, when menstruation finally ceases. Most women experience some menopausal symptoms, which are caused by declining production of the female hormone oestrogen. These include irregular periods, hot flushes, frequent headaches, weight gain, dry vaginal tissue, cystitis, depression and insomnia. Without the calcium-holding effect of oestrogen, bone mass is gradually diminished and the hormonal protection against heart disease ceases. The menopause is a difficult time for women both physically and psychologically, so partners and families should try to be supportive.

A healthy diet, regular exercise, sufficient sleep, relaxation and mental stimulation help menopausal women retain a happy and positive attitude to life. Hormone replacement therapy (HRT) alleviates the worst of physical symptoms like vaginal dryness and hot flushes, but is not suitable for all women.

Certain natural substances also improve a woman's wellbeing at this time: these include homoeopathic remedies *Glonoine* and *Lachesis* ; aromatherapy with essential oils of *sage, cypress* and *geranium*; herbal infusions or teas made with *lime-blossom* or *camomile,* and *passiflora* tablets. Branded menopausal supplements are also available from health food stores and pharmacies.

Solgar have recently launched some innovative new products based on phytoestrogens (plant hormones). These have been specifically developed to enhance the health of menopausal women.

Osteoporosis

A condition in which the bones become progressively thinner, weaker and more brittle, due mainly to loss of calcium. Bones naturally become less dense as we age, but in osteoporosis the thinning is more progressive.

Post-menopausal women are the main sufferers, as their bones no longer benefit from the calcium-holding benefits of oestrogen. Although the tendency to osteoporosis is inherited, strong bones can be built up by eating a healthy diet with a good calcium intake and not smoking. Taking regular exercise throughout life is also important, as this improves blood flow and increases bone density.

'At risk' patients are offered a bone density scan and prescribed hormone replacement therapy (HRT), the standard conventional treatment for osteoporosis.

Premenstrual Syndrome

About 40 percent of women suffer premenstrual symptoms of one kind or another. These are caused by a change in the balance of female hormones during the menstrual cycle, increasing water and salt in the system, and a shortage of progesterone. Lack of essential fatty acids, a deficiency of certain minerals and vitamin B6 are known to aggravate the varied symptoms of PMS, which include weight gain, mood swings, irritability and food and alcohol cravings.

Effective well-tried natural remedies for PMS include evening primrose oil with vitamin B6, the herbal remedy *agnus castus* and a magnesium supplement such as *Magnesium OK* – all available from health food stores and pharmacies.

Seasonal Affective Disorder *(SAD)*

A newly recognised illness caused by a lack of sunlight and affecting people living in countries where winter brings short daylight hours and long dark evenings. It causes varying degrees of depression and fatigue over the winter months. The condition can be dramatically improved or even cured by spending a few hours a day in front of a special lightbox. The shortened hours of daylight are replaced with artificial light specially designed to mimic sunlight, a treatment known as phototherapy. SAD is quickly cured by phototherapy, which eases the depression and enables sufferers to become more energetic, motivated and sociable.

New research into SAD suggests that extracts of the herb hypericum (also known as St John's wort) show promising results as an alternative treatment for those who find light therapy too time-consuming or do not want to take antidepressant drugs like *Prozac*. Hypericum has long been used as a natural treatment for depression, and is believed to work on the brain's neurotransmitter chemical serotonin (as do the new antidepressants), but with fewer side-effects.

Stress

Long-term stress takes its toll mentally and physically, causing a wide range of health symptoms including raised blood pressure, depression, panic attacks, digestive and skin disorders, headaches and insomnia. The body's reaction to a stressful situation is to produce extra hormones and these further increase the anxiety state.

Many alternative treatments offer stress management and help in overcoming anxiety and emotional blocks: Yoga, aromatherapy, hydrotherapy, biofeedback, dance movement and polarity therapy have especially good techniques for unwinding and relaxation; psychotherapy and counselling enable the sufferer to find the cause of the stress and advise on how to reduce or overcome it.

Thrush

A common and unpleasant affliction caused when the *Candida albicans* fungus, a yeast-like organism that normally inhabits the bowel, becomes overactive and spreads into other body areas. Thrush is particularly likely to occur when the immune system is below par, due to stress, illness or hormonal changes. The candida organism thrives in warm, moist areas of the body like the mouth and vagina, causing discomfort and itching, often with white flaking skin exposing sore red areas underneath.

A course of antibiotics may trigger an attack of thrush, as the drugs kill the friendly gut bacteria that keep the candida organism under control. Taking a garlic supplement after a course of antibiotics is a wise precaution, as it helps restore normal bowel flora and prevents a candida overgrowth.

Candida infections should be diagnosed and treated quickly, as the organism may spread and cause many chronic and vague symptoms of ill-health, especially digestive problems.

Orthodox medical treatment for thrush includes lotions, creams, ointments, pessaries and oral preparations to suppress the symptoms. Alternative treatment aims to stop overgrowth of the micro-organism, which means cutting out sugar and refined starches (on which the yeast thrives) and eating more wholefoods. Garlic and acidophilus supplements will suppress excess fungal growth and restore the balance of micro-organisms in the gut.

Frequent salt water washes and the application of live natural yoghurt are helpful in vaginal thrush. Strict attention to personal hygiene is also important. Both sexual partners must be treated for the infection even if only one has symptoms. Anyone prone to thrush should avoid bubble baths, tampons, strong detergents and tight or nylon underwear, as they are likely to make the condition worse.

Tinnitus

A distressing condition causing hissing, whistling or ringing sounds in one or both ears. It is usually associated with damage to the inner ear and some degree of deafness.

Various drugs are prescribed for the condition, and some sufferers obtain relief by covering the tinnitus noises with personal headphones or white noise generators (tinnitus maskers).

The alternative therapies cranial osteopathy, biofeedback relaxation techniques and acupressure may help tinnitus. A supplement of ginkgo biloba is also recommended, as the herb improves circulation and blood flow to the head and brain and has important antioxidant properties.

It may also be a good idea to consult with a nutritionally-trained doctor to check that the inner ear problems are not caused by a deficiency of vitamin A, vitamin D, iron or zinc. Sometimes tinnitus is helped by extra intakes of magnesium, potassium and manganese.

Suggested essential oils for different needs

Cellulite	Cypress, geranium, rosemary, sage, neroli, pine
Colds	Eucalyptus, pine, thyme, peppermint, camphor, myrrh, neroli
Cystitis	Sandalwood, lavender, cypress
Digestive problems	Parsley, cardamom, marjoram, cinnamon, mugwort, peppermint orange, verbena
Eczema	Thyme, camomile, patchouli
Menopause	Cypress
Menstrual problems	Sandalwood, rose, verbena, mugwort
Relaxation	Rosewood, lavender, cinnamon, cedarwood
Sensuality	Ylang ylang, sandalwood, bergamot, cedarwood, lavender
Spots	Geranium, jojoba oil, sandalwood, rose
Stress and tension	Camomile, lavender, juniper, bergamot, neroli, thyme, sandalwood
Vitality	Rosemary, juniper, grapefruit, lemongrass, lime, bergamot

PART THREE

Spa Therapies and Beauty Treatments

The growing interest in alternative medicine emphasises the importance of a healthy diet and lifestyle. This means not only taking regular exercise, but allowing time for rest and relaxation, a philosophy the health resorts have been following for years.

Now, these peaceful retreats are enjoying a fresh wave of popularity, with many resorts expanding and refurbishing to keep pace with the demand for their services. The combination of treatments, healthy food, and a varied range of exercise facilities, is proving an irresistible attraction to busy folk needing some time for themselves, to unwind and revitalise.

Although new treatments are offered every year, facials, massage and aromatherapy continue to be the most sought after forms of pampering.

Spa and recreational facilities have also been added to many hotels and leisure clubs, but for most people, a weekend at a dedicated health resort is the ultimate short break.

Aromatherapy

An enjoyable and therapeutic pressure point massage using essential oils with various helpful properties. A selection of oils are chosen specifically for each client after an initial consultation with the therapist.

Aromazone Therapy

A lymphatic massage to improve circulation and reduce fluid retention and toxins in the body. Air pressure is used to inflate and deflate specially designed leggings and sleeves which exert a gentle, intermittent counter pressure around the limbs. The treatment speeds lymph flow, eliminates water retention and releases toxic waste matter from the tissues. This effective and energising treatment is best taken as a course of four to six sessions.

Bleaching

A beauty treatment that temporarily camouflages superfluous hair by lightening it to blend in with the skin tone. Different bleach solutions are used on different parts of the body. Bleaching is favoured by those who cannot face the discomfort of other types of hair removal.

Blitz Jet Douche

A popular thalassotherapy (sea water) body treatment from France now offered at many health resorts worldwide. The recipient stands in a tiled area and is massaged from a distance of about three metres, by a powerful jet of warmed water from a hose. The therapist massages the entire body from the soles of the feet up to the neck and shoulders using this hose, – finishing with an optional cold water spray. This exhilarating treatment stimulates the circulation and helps eliminate toxins from the body.

Body Scrub/Exfoliation

A treatment recommended on its own or as a preparation for other body treatments or tanning. After showering, a slightly abrasive paste is applied to the limbs and body. A few minutes later, this is massaged or showered away leaving the skin soft and clean. A body scrub or exfoliation is a quick and invigorating way to remove dead cells and improve the overall appearance of the skin.

Body/Seaweed /Herbal Wrap

A wonderfully relaxing and pampering treatment in which the body is covered in various oils and gels. The recipient is then wrapped in a sheet steamed in aromatic herbs, covered with a light blanket and left to relax in this pleasantly warm environment for about twenty minutes. The treatment helps to remove toxins and excess fluid from the body.

Bust Treatment

Bust treatments are as common in France as facials, but tend to be less popular elsewhere. They may be offered at salons and health resorts that use French beauty products or Cathiodermie (see next entry).

The treatment usually consists of a skin exfoliation followed by the application of specialised products and massage. Bust treatments are designed to tone, firm and strengthen the skin, helping to improve bust shape. They cannot reduce or increase the size of the bust, but a course of treatments should make the skin look smoother and improve skin tone.

Cathiodermie

A facial and body treatment devised by French cosmetic chemist Rene Guinot, which uses mild electrical currents to deep cleanse the skin. This oxygenates the outer skin layer, improving its texture and encouraging regeneration. A Cathiodermie facial treatment includes a face mask and lasts about ninety minutes. Cathiodermie treatments can also be used on other parts of the body.

As Cathiodermie cleanses so thoroughly, the skin must be allowed time to recover, so sunbathing and make up should be avoided immediately after a treatment. The skin may also become a bit spotty, as all the impurities have been brought to the surface. After a few days when these clear up, the skin should look in great condition. The deep cleansing properties of Cathiodermie make it a particularly good treatment for anyone suffering from acne.

Because the treatment uses a mild electrical current, Cathiodermie is not recommended for anyone fitted with a pacemaker or suffering from epilepsy.

Cleortherm

A heat treatment for the body which improves the circulation and helps remove cellulite. Cleortherm is similar to a herbal wrap except that, after covering the body in essential oils and gels, the recipient is wrapped in a specially insulated electric blanket and left to sweat profusely for about 30 minutes. During the treatment, up to 1.5kg/3lbs of body fluid may be eliminated.

Cleortherm treatments are quite exacting, so should not be taken during pregnancy or by anyone with diabetes or high or low blood pressure.

Cryosurgery

A process offered in specialist beauty salons, using local freezing to remove unwanted or abnormal tissue from the skin and mucous membranes. It quickly and effectively removes skin tags, warts and other bumps and lumps on the skin of the face and body. Discomfort is minimal and healing should leave no scars.

Dry Floatation

A totally relaxing experience which involves floating (without getting wet) on a specially constructed water mattress. It provides ideal relaxation for those who find ordinary floatation too chilly or claustrophobic. So that the experience is as restful and enjoyable as possible, the lights are turned down and gentle music is played.

Health resorts offering this treatment may combine a dry float with a mud or hay bath or a body wrap.

Electrolysis

A method of permanently removing unwanted hair from the face and body, using an electronically charged needle applied to the hair root. Different types of electrolysis include a mix of galvanic and short-wave diathermy, known as the Blend. There is also the (Sylvia Lewis) Method, which uses a specially designed rigid L-shaped needle and a more moderated current. Disposable needles should always be used.

Because each hair has to be removed separately, electrolysis is an expensive and time-consuming process that may also be uncomfortable. Its success depends on the skill of the therapist. Electrolysis is especially good for removing facial hairs, and can also be used to treat fine thread veins.

Exfoliation

A facial or body treatment which removes dead skin cells by applying salt or an abrasive lotion. This cleanses and softens the skin and invigorates the body. Recommended on its own or as a preparation for tanning.

Eyelash and Eyebrow tinting

Eyelash and eyebrow tinting is used to temporarily darken the lashes and brows to give them better definition. The tints used are similar to hair dyes, but more gentle, and the effects last for several weeks.

Eyelash tinting is an ideal beauty treatment to have prior to a holiday, as it eliminates the need for mascara (unless thicker eyelashes are desired).

Facial

The most popular treatment in the beauty salon. The face and neck are thoroughly cleansed, toned and moisturised using products suited to individual skin conditions and types.

Many different types of facials are available, some with strangely non-descriptive names like *Paris* and *Hollywood*. Facials for every type of skin condition are offered by leading salons and health resorts, varying from deep cleansing treatments to help teenage spots to rejuvenating collagen for mature skins. The beauty therapist can explain the choices offered and advise on suitability.

Fango/Parafango Therapy

A soothing heat treatment used extensively in European spas. Mineralised or volcanic mud is mixed with spa water and other components to the consistency of modelling clay. This is heated and used as a poultice to cover joints and areas of the body affected by arthritis or other painful conditions. The pack retains the heat for at least 30 minutes, enabling the warmth and healing components of the mud to be absorbed through the skin. A series of treatments is usually prescribed for effective and natural pain relief.

Faradic Exercise

Slendertone is the most well-known form of faradic treatment – a passive electrically-controlled muscle stimulation designed to tone and firm the body.

Soft rubber pads with self-adhesive straps are attached to areas of the body that need toning up. A low voltage electrical current is then switched on causing a mild tingling sensation which encourages the muscles to contract. For the most effective treatment, all 16 pads should be used with the strongest tolerable intensity of current. Some firming of the body and inch loss will be noticeable after a series of regular 30 or 45 minute sessions.

Floatation

Floatation has become a popular way of relaxing and floatation tanks are now found in many health clubs and health resorts. During a session, which lasts about an hour, the client floats effortlessly in an enclosed tank of shallow warm water, in which Epsom salts and other minerals have been dissolved. Donning a bathing cap (or using a head support) and applying vaseline to any nicks or cuts on the skin will make the float more comfortable. When the client is ready, the lights are turned down so that the floating can be carried out in the dark. Although the purpose of a float is total relaxation and the absence of sensory awareness, some floatation centres play relaxing taped music. When there are no distractions like light, outside noises or the water being too cool, a profound level of relaxation may be achieved. Having a float after a long flight is a great way to overcome jet lag.

Floatation is a totally unique experience and not at all claustrophobic – the tank is never locked and the client can finish the float at any time.

G5 Massage

A deep gyratory massage treatment using various electrically-driven applicator heads (five originally, hence the name G5) on different parts of the body. This is a powerful and effective treatment for tension or fatigue and it also tones the body. G5 has a much stronger effect than a massage given by hand.

Galvanic Treatment

A slimming treatment to tone and firm areas of the body, often used in conjunction with faradic treatments like *Slendertone*. The low-voltage galvanic current encourages the absorption of liquids into the skin via current-conducting clay and electrodes. These are placed on the body areas that require to be tightened and firmed, as in *Ionithermie* treatments.

A one-off treatment can achieve a temporary size reduction Several treatments will have a more lasting effect, but unless dieting is undertaken at the same time, the improvement will not be permanent.

Hellerwork

An American therapy designed to restore the body's balance, returning it to a relaxed and more youthful state by releasing built-up tensions and stress. Hellerwork combines manipulation of connective body tissue with discussion on the effects of emotions and mental attitudes on the body. It helps to increase awareness of movements that keep the body supple and tension-free.

Infra-Red

A heat treatment using infra-red light to heal painful muscles and body aches. The client lies on a treatment couch and special infra-red lamps are placed over the affected area. The warming infra red light helps the muscles relax and increases circulation of blood, which in turn promotes self-healing Infra-red treatments are often used with physiotherapy to ease sports injuries.

Karwendel

A European spa treatment using fossil oils to relax and refresh the body. The thick, tarry substance is rich in nutrients and is added to a warm, therapeutic bath, to stimulate the circulation and help clear up problem skin.

Karwendel treatments are particularly beneficial to sufferers of psoriasis and other skin conditions.

Kneipp Therapy

A cold water treatment used extensively in Germany and Austria. It works through the reaction of the body to cold stimulation, improving metabolism and blood supply and strengthening the nervous system.

The treatment takes several days and consists of body packs, cold water wraps, dieting and a system of alternating 'dry' and 'drinking' days. The aim is to detoxify the whole body which is relieved of excess water and fat.

Kneipp therapy is not as unpleasant as it sounds and the client's progress is carefully monitored at every stage. All body packs and cold water wraps are applied in the comfort of a warm private room.

Manicure

A beauty treatment for the hands to make the nails look healthy and attractive. A basic manicure includes the application of various creams and lotions to cleanse, massage and nourish the skin and nails. The softened cuticles are gently pushed back, and the nails are painted using a basecoat, several coats of varnish and a top coat. For best results the varnish should be allowed to dry naturally.

Some health resorts and salons offer luxury manicures incorporating massage and moisturising treatments to improve the condition of the hands.

Massage

A body massage is one of life's special treats. Swedish massage is the type of body massage most commonly offered at spas and health resorts. It uses long sweeping movements interspersed with kneading and pummelling. Fatigue and tension are massaged away with the help of scented oils to reduce friction. An enjoyable and rejuvenating treatment for everyone.

Moor Peat Bath

A spa treatment recommended for rheumatism sufferers. A mixture of liquid peat is add to a warm bath. The nutrients and mineral salts in the peat create a soothing and therapeutic effect. The treatment ends with a rest in a warm room.

Mud Therapy

Certain muds are acknowledged to have health-giving properties. They are a rich source of nutrients from dissolved minerals and plant substances, accumulated over thousands of years. Some are used therapeutically in the form of mud baths, mud packs and packaged mud products. Mud from Austria's *Neydharting* spa contains natural antibiotics and large quantities of minerals and vitamins, while *Dead Sea* mud and mineral treatments are renowned for treating skin diseases like psoriasis and eczema. *Parafango* (also called *fango*) is a hot volcanic mud from Padua in Italy, which is mixed with a wax and then applied like a poultice. It is used to treat painful joints and arthritis.

The drying, abrasive action of mud on the skin has a cleansing and invigorating effect on the whole body. Although clinically unproven, beneficial substances in the mud are thought to be absorbed through the skin into the bloodstream and circulation. Tiny nerve fibres in the outer layers of the skin are also stimulated, benefiting the whole nervous system.

Most therapeutic spas, health resorts and specialist beauty salons offer mud treatments.

Needle Shower

An overhead shower with additional water outlets placed at different body levels to give a horizontal spray massage. Pleasantly invigorating.

Panthermal

An enjoyable body treatment that thoroughly cleanses and tones the skin. The client climbs into a specially constructed domed steam cabinet and lies on a wooden slatted rack, keeping the head outside. The dome fills up with vapour which opens the pores of the skin and causes profuse sweating (the cabinet temperature remains around 38°C. throughout, so the body never gets too hot). Then the cabinet fills up with oxygen to rejuvenate and freshen the skin. After this, a blend of selected essential oils is sprayed into the cabinet. The treatment ends with a cool needle-jet shower to pep up the circulation and close the pores.

This is a refreshing treatment lasting about 30 minutes and is not as exhausting as the steam cabinet. Available at some health resorts and large beauty salons.

Paraffin Wax Baths

Not a bath to immerse in! A thick layer of warm wax is brushed all over the body, which is wrapped up in waxproof paper and covered with a towel to retain the heat. As the body perspires, the heat draws out the toxins, cleansing the pores and softening the skin.

Paraffin wax is also used as a localised treatment for the hands and feet. It relieves the pain of arthritis and stiff joints and has the added bonus of softening the skin.

Pedicure

A truly pampering treatment with long lasting benefits. The feet are first immersed in warm water or a footbath to soften the skin and nails, then dried and moisturised. The toenails are trimmed and the nail cuticles gently pushed back. Hardened skin on the heels and soles is buffed away, leaving the feet smooth and soft. After this, the toenails are varnished with several coats of polish. Some luxury pedicures also include leg and foot massage.

Rolfing

A vigorous massage technique created by American biochemist Ida Rolf. It is used to realign the body by manipulating the connective tissue covering the muscles and organs, and can also be applied (gently) to the face to improve circulation and muscle tone.

Salt Rub

A brisk body rub given after showering. Salt is massaged all over the body by hand or with a loofah then rinsed off. Salt rubs are often given prior to a hydrotherapy massage bath and are very invigorating, leaving the skin soft and glowing.

Sauna

A popular dry heat treatment originating from Finland, where it is traditionally followed with a birch twig massage and a roll in the snow! A sauna is usually taken in a wood-lined room or cabin complete with wooden benches for sitting or reclining. Burning coals create a hot, dry atmosphere and a temperature between 40°C and 80°C.

Saunas are best taken wearing nothing but a towel or swimsuit, as the heat induces profuse sweating and encourages the removal of toxins and waste products through the pores of the skin. Regular saunas soothe aching joints and stimulate the circulation.

Building up tolerance to the dry heat is a gradual process. Most people find five to ten minutes at first is long enough. The treatment ends with a cool shower or cold plunge to close the pores. A short rest should be taken after any heat treatment to allow body temperature and blood pressure to return to normal.

Saunas should not be taken by pregnant women, or anyone with high or low blood pressure, diabetes or heart problems.

Sclerotherapy

A treatment for thread veins – the fine broken veins

commonly found on the legs and face. A diluted form of a drug used on varicose veins is injected into the broken thread veins. This causes the veins to shrink, pushing blood out of the tissues and causing a bruise. As the bruise is gradually re-absorbed, the broken veins also disappear.

Scottish Douche

A shower of alternating hot and cold water jets to stimulate the spinal column and tone up the circulation and nervous system. Usually found in therapeutic European spas.

Sitz Bath

A hydrotherapy treatment taken in a hipbath with two parts, one filled with hot water the other cold. The person undergoing the treatment sits for a few minutes in the hot water with feet in the cold water, then alternates the process. This effective natural treatment is used in therapeutic spas to improve circulation, and as an aid in prostate and some gynaecological conditions.

Steam Bath

A popular heat treatment to promote sweating and remove body toxins. Like the sauna, the steam room also has shelving for relaxing. Menthol vapours may be added to aid inhalation. Many people find the wet heat of the steam room more tolerable than the dry heat of the sauna.

Steam Cabinet

The steam cabinet offers a more intense detox treatment than the steam room, but is pleasant and relaxing at the same time. The length of treatment depends on the stamina of the recipient, but is usually about 15 – 25 minutes. Unlike the steam room, the head remains outside the cabinet and is not exposed to the heat, while the rest of the body sweats profusely inside. The steam cabinet is more intense than a steam room and is offered as a treatment at many health resorts and spas. Best followed by a 30 minute relaxation and a body massage.

Thai Massage

Like other oriental therapies, Thai massage is based on the concept of energy flow through the meridian lines of the body. Thai massage concentrates on the meridian lines themselves rather than the pressure points. To undertake the massage, the client lies fully clothed on a mat on the floor. A massage involves a lot of leg work, with the therapist stretching and bending the client's limbs. Thai massage tends to be quite vigorous, but relaxing at the same time. It is particularly good for stress-related disorders, lower back pain and headaches.

Thalassotherapy

The therapeutic use of sea water, seaweeds and other marine components. Used in hydrotherapy treatments and baths, showers, sprays, seaweed wraps and facials. Thalassotherapy is traditionally French. Many centres are based on the invigorating Atlantic coast, where the health-giving properties of the marine environment are fully exploited.

Thalassotherapy's worldwide popularity has led to the development of dried products and muds for use at inland health resorts and spas. Pleasant as they are, such treatments cannot be classed as authentic thalassotherapy as they do not use real sea water.

Turkish Bath

Genuine Turkish baths are a series of increasingly hot and humid steam rooms complete with marble slabs for resting as the body sweats profusely. When the hottest steam room is reached, the journey is reversed so that the body has a chance to cool down, before the session finishes with a cool shower and a rest.

Steam rooms and cabinets work on the same principle, but cannot be compared with genuine Turkish baths. Many people find steam a more tolerable heat treatment than sauna – both are equally effective in removing body toxins and waste through the pores of the skin.

The English spa town of Harrogate offers visitors a splendid example of a fully operating Turkish bath.

Underwater Massage

Massage given in a warm bath by high pressure jets of water within the bath, to which peat or seaweed may be added. The process helps to break down cellulite and improve the circulation, but is not suitable for anyone who bruises easily or has raised blood pressure. Underwater massage can also be given by a therapist with a hand-held, high pressure hose. This is a strong and therapeutic treatment.

Waxing

The removal of unwanted hair from the body, legs and face using a warm wax thinly applied. Muslin strips are pressed onto the waxed hairs, which are then swiftly pulled out. Waxing is more successful than shaving, as re-growths are much slower and softer. As the hair grows back with a fine end not a blunt one, there is no unsightly stubble.

PART FOUR

Alternative Medicine Registers and Associations

Many of these organisations have limited resources and may be difficult to contact. It is probably best to write for further details (always enclose a sae) or be prepared to leave a message on an answering machine.

Acupuncture

British Council for Acupuncture
BCA, Park House, 206-208 Latimer Road,
London W10 6RE
Tel 0181-964 0222 Fax 0181-964 0333
1500 members use MBAcC after their name, Send sae for local practitioner or £3.50 cheque/postal order for full register

British Medical Acupuncture Society
BMAS, Newton House, Newton Lane, Whitley,
Warrington, WA4 4JA
Tel 01925 730727 Fax 01925 730492
1350 medically qualified practitioners

Society of Auricular Acupuncture
SAA, Nurstead Lodge, Nurstead, Meopham,
Kent DA13 9AD
Tel 01474 813902 Fax 01474 813770
60 members(MSAAc.) Send A4 sae for list of practitioners using electro-acupuncture rather than needles

Alexander Technique

Society of Teachers of Alexander Technique
STAT, 266 Fulham Road, London SW10 9EL
Tel 0171-351 0828 Fax 0171-352 1556
714 members

Alexander Technique International
ATI, Ewen Villa, Villiers Street, Hyde,
Cheshire, SK14 2SA
Tel 0161 368 9719
46 members

Aromatherapy

Aromatherapy Organisations Council
AOC, 3 Latymer Close, Braybrooke, Market
Harborough, Leicestershire LE16 8LN
Tel/fax 01858 434242
6000 members

Association of Medical Aromatherapists
AMA, 11 Park Circus, Glasgow G3 6AX
Tel 0141 332 4924 Fax 0141 353 3783
Approximately 100 members

Art Therapy

Arts Therapy Association,
c/o Arts Therapy Department, Springfield Hospital,
61 Glenburnie Road, London SW17 7DJ.
Postal enquiries only

Autogenic Therapy

British Association for Autogenic Training
and Therapy
BAFATT c/o Royal London Homoeopathic Hospital,
Great Ormond St, London WC1N 3HR
86 members
Postal enquiries only

Ayurveda

Ayurvedic Living
PO Box 188, Exeter, Devon, EX4 5AY
(send sae for details & practitioners)

Maharishi Ayur-Veda Health Centres UK
For nationwide network of centres send sae to:
Freepost, WN5 1037, Skelmersdale, Lancashire WN8
6BR Tel 0990 143733

Bates Eye Method

Bates Association of Great Britain
PO Box 25, Shoreham by Sea, West Sussex BN43 6ZF
Send £1 and sae for register & information

BiomagnetiC Therapy

The British Biomagnetic Association
The Williams Clinic, 31 St Marychurch Road,
Torquay, Devon TQ1 3JF
Tel 01803 293346
218 members (MBBA) For local practitioner details send sae

Chiropractic

British Chiropractic Association
BCA, Blagrave House, 17 Blagrave Street, Reading,
Berks, RG1 1QB
Tel 0118 9505950 Fax 0118 9588946
750 members

McTimoney Chiropractic Association
McTCA, 21 High Street, Eynsham, Oxford OX8 1HE
Tel 01865 880974 Fax 01865 880975
300 members

Colonic Irrigation

Colonic International Association
16 Englands Lane, London NW3 4TG
Tel/fax 0171-483 1595
Send A4 sae for register

Counselling

British Association for Counselling (BAC)
1 Regent Place, Rugby, Warwickshire CV21 2PJ
Tel 01788 550899

Craniosacral Therapy

The Craniosacral Therapy Association
CTA, 27 Old Gloucester St, London WC1N 3XX
Tel 0181-543 4969

The Upledger Institute 52 Main Street, Perth, PH2 7HB
Tel 01738 444404

Crystal Therapy

Affiliation of Crystal Healing Organisations
46 Lower Green Road, Esher, Surrey KT10 8HD
Tel 0181-398 7252
50 members
Send A5 sae for details

International Association of Crystal Healing Therapists
Unit 24-26 The Coliseum, Church Street, Manchester M4 1PN
Tel 0161 702 8191
Send large sae for list of practitioners

Dance Movement/Art Therapy

Arts Therapy Association,
c/o Arts Therapy Department, Springfield Hospital,
61 Glenburnie Road, London SW17 7DJ.
(postal enquiries only)

Feldenkrais Method

The Feldenkrais Guild UK
Tel 07000 785 506

Floatation

For a list of centres with tanks contact
The Floatation Tank Association
PO Box 11024, London SW4 7ZF
Tel 0171-627 4962

The Float Information Service
Tel 0171-357 0302

Flower Remedies (Bach)

The Bach Centre,
Mount Vernon, Sotwell, Wallingford,
Oxfordshire OX10 0PZ
Tel 01491 834678
300 practitioners

Healing

The Confederation of Healing Organisations
113 High Street, Berkhamstead, HP4 2DJ
15 organisations of qualified healers.
Send first class sae

National Federation of Spiritual Healers
Old Manor Farm Studio, Church Street,
Sunbury-on-Thames, Middlesex TW16 6RG
Tel 0891 616080

Hellerwork

Information on receipt of a sae sent to:
Suite 211, Coppergate House, 16 Brune Street,
London E1 7NJ

Herbal Medicine

National Institute of Medical Herbalists
56 Longbrook Street, Exeter, Devon, EX4 6AH
Tel 01392 426022
295 members (MNIMH or FNIMH) Send large sae and 31p stamp for register

Homoeopathy

Society of Homoeopaths
2 Artisan Road, Northampton, NN1 4HU
Tel 01604 21400
500 practitioner members (RSHom or FSHom) Send large sae for register

The Homoeopathic Trust (The Homoeopathic Society) Hahnemann House, 2 Powis Place, Great Ormond Street, London WC1N 3HT
Tel 0171-837 9469
Represents only medically qualified homoeopaths. Send sae for a list of NHS and private practitioners

UK Homoeopathic Medical Association
2 Livingstone Road, Gravesend, Kent DA12 5DZ
Tel/fax 01474 560336
380 members MHM(UK)

Hypnotherapy/Psychotherapy

The National Register of Hypnotherapists and Psychotherapists
12 Cross Street, Nelson, Lancashire, BB9 7EN
Tel 01282 699378
345 members (MNRHP)

UK Council for Psychology
UKCP, 167-169 Great Portland St, London W1N 5FB
Tel 0171-436 3002
Approved therapists use letters UKCP
Telephone for details

Iridology

Guild of Naturopathic Iridologists
94 Grosvenor Road, London SW1V 3LF
Tel 0171-834 3579
52 practitioners

International Association of Clinical Iridologists
853 Finchley Road, London NW11 8LX
30 practitioners

Kinesiology

Association for Systemic Kinesiology
39 Browns Road, Surbiton, Surrey KT5 8ST
Tel 0181-399 3215
200 members

The Kinesiology Federation
KF, PO Box 83 Sheffield, South Yorkshire S7 2YN
Tel/fax 0114 281 4064
Umbrella organisation representing
200 practitioners.
Send sae for local practitioners and details

Kirlian Photography

Association of Kirlian Practitioners
c/o Guy Mason
Tel 01730 821690

Macrobiotics

Macrobiotic Association of Great Britain
The Tardis, 34 Banbury Road, Ettington,
Stratford-upon-Avon, Warwickshire CV37 7SU

Magnetic Therapy

British Biomagnetic Association
31 St Marychurch Road, Torquay, Devon, TQ1 3JF
Tel 01803 293346

Manual Lymphatic Drainage

MLD UK
PO Box 149, Wallingford, Oxfordshire OX10 7LD
75 members

Massage

British Massage Therapy Council
Greenbank House, 65a Adelphi Street, Preston,
Lancashire, PR1 7BH
Tel 01772 881063
603 members

Scottish Massage Therapists Organisation
70 Lochside Road, Denmore Park, Bridge of Don,
Aberdeen AB23 8QW
Tel 01224 822960
312 members

Metamorphic Technique

Metamorphic Association
67 Ritherdon Road, London SW17 8QE

Naturopathy

General Council & Register of Naturopaths
Goswell House, 2 Goswell Road, Street,
Somerset BA16 0JG
Tel 01458 840072
236 members NaD MRN
Send sae and £2.50 cheque for details

Nutritional Therapy

Society for Promotion of Nutritional Therapy
PO Box 47, Heathfield, East Sussex, TN21 8ZX
Tel 01825 872921
800 members

The Institute of Optimum Nutrition
Blades Court, Deodar Road, London SW15 2NU
Tel 0181 877 9993

British Society for Allergy, Environmental and
Nutritional Medicine
PO Box 28, Totton, Southampton,
Hampshire, SO40 2ZA
Can supply a list of private doctors interested in nutrition and food allergies

Osteopathy

Osteopathic Information Service
PO Box 2074, Reading, Berkshire RG1 4YR
Tel 0118 9512051
Represents 2800 practitioners

General Council and Register of Osteopaths
GCRO, 56 London Street, Reading, Berks RG1 4SQ
Tel 0118 957 6585
Fax 0118 956 6246
1850 members

Pilates

The Pilates Foundation
5 Harrington Road, London SW7 3ES
Tel 07071-781859
Send large sae for details and local classes
Pilates Off the Square
Tel 0171-495 0374
Pilates classes in London area

Polarity Therapy

United Kingdom Polarity Therapy Association
Monomark House, 27 Old Gloucester Street,
London WC1N 3XX
Tel 01483 417714
80 members

Radionics

The Confederation of Radionic Organisations,
Maperton Trust, Maperton, Wincanton, Somerset, BA9 8EH
Tel 01963 32651

Reiki

The Reiki Association
Mel Jones, Cornbrook Bridge House, Clee Hill,
Ludlow, Shropshire SY8 3QQ
Tel 01980 550829

Reflexology/Zone Therapy

Association of Reflexologists
27 Old Gloucester Street, London, WC1N 3XX
Tel 0990 673320
3870 members (MAR)

British Reflexology Association
BRA , Monks Orchard, Whitbourne,
Worcester WR6 5RB
Tel/fax 01886 8211207
700 members (MBRA)

International Federation of Reflexologists
76/78 Eldridge Road, Croydon, Surrey CR0 1EF
Tel 0181-667 9458
1200 members (MIFR)

Rolfing

For further information call 0171-834 1493

Shiatsu

The Shiatsu Society
Interchange Studios, Dalby Street,
London NW5 3NQ
Tel 0171-813 7772 Fax 0171-813 7773
430 members

Traditional Chinese Medicine

Register of Chinese Herbal Medicine
RCHM, PO Box 400, Wembley, Middlesex HA9 9NZ
Tel 0171-224 0883 Fax 0171-377 8553
250 members
Send sae and £2.50 cheque or postal order

Yoga

The British Wheel of Yoga
1 Hamilton Place, Boston Road, Sleaford,
Lincolnshire NG34 7ES
Tel 01529 306851

Other Useful Addresses

British Complementary Medicine Association
BCMA, 249 Sosse Road, Leicester LE3 1AE
Tel 0116 2825511

Council for Complementary and Alternative Medicine
CCAM, Park House, 206 - 208 Latimer Road, London W10 6RE
Tel 0181-968 3862

The Institute for Complementary Medicine
ICM, PO Box 194, London SE16 1QZ
Tel 0171-237 5165
Fax 0171-237 5175
(send sae with three first class stamps)

Arts Therapy Association
c/o Arts Therapy Department, Springfield Hospital,
61 Glenburnie Road, London SW17 7DJ

The Council for Nutrition Education and Therapy
CNEAT, 1 The Close, Halton, Aylesbury, Buckinghamshire HP22 5NJ

British Spas Federation
BSF, Mount Carlees, Ruan Major, Helston, Cornwall, TR12 7LL
Tel/fax 01326 290391

The Health Education Authority
HEA, Hamilton House, Mabledon Place, London WC1H 9TX
Tel 0171-383 3833

Dead Sea Mud Treatments
Bharti Vyas
Advice helpline and mail order service,
Tel 0171-486 7910.

Medicur
Portable magnetic field device for treatment of pain. For further details,
tel 0115 914 1144.

Seasonal Affective
Disorder (SAD)
Association
PO Box 989, Steyning,
West Sussex BN44 3HG
*Send £5 cheque for
information pack*

British Association of
Homoeopathic
Veterinary Surgeons
Chinham House,
Stanford-in the Vale,
Faringdon, Oxon
SN7 8NQ
Send sae for diagnosis

British Homoeopathic
Dental Association
12 Wellington Road,
Watford, Herts
WD1 1QW
*150 practitioners
Send sae for details*

International Register of
Holistic Therapists
(Beauty, reflexology,
massage)
38a Portsmouth Road,
Woolston, Southampton
Hants, SO19 9AD
Tel 01703 422695
*Send £4 for details and
register*

The UK T'Ai Chi
Association
PO Box 159, Bromley,
Kent BR1 3XX
Tel 0181-289 5166
Send sae for detail

Specialist Spa Travel Agents

Erna Low Ltd
9 Reece Mews, London
SW7 3HE
Tel 0171-584 2841
Free brochure

Thermalia Travel Ltd
12 New College Parade,
Finchley Road, Swiss
Cottage, London
NW3 5EP
Tel 0171-483 1898
Free brochure

INDEX

A

Acne	43
Acupuncture	09
Acupressure	09
Addresses	75
Alexander Technique	10
Allergy	44
Aromatherapy	10, 60
Aromazone Therapy	60
Art Therapy	11
Arthritis	44
Autogenic Training	11
Ayurvedic Medicine	12

B

Bach Flower Remedies	12
Balneotherapy	13
Bates Eye Method	13
Biochemics	14
Biofeedback	14
Biomagnetic Therapy	15
Blitz Jet Douche	60
Body Scrub	61
Body Wrap	61
Breast Pain	45
Bust Treatment	61

C

Cathiodermie	62
Cellulite	46
Chiropractic	15
Chronic Fatigue Syndrome	46
Cleortherm	62
Clinical Ecology	16
Clinical Nutrition	16
Cold Sores	47
Colonic Irrigation	17
Colour Therapy	17
Counselling	18
Cranial Massage	19
Craniosacral Therapy	19
Cryosurgery	63
Crystal Therapy	19
Cystitis	48

D

Dance Therapy	20
Depression	49
Dowsing	20
Dry Floatation	63

E

Electrolysis	63
Electrotherapy	20
Eczema	50
Exfoliation	64
Eyelash Tinting	64

F
- Facial 64
- Fango Therapy 64
- Faradic Exercise 65
- Fasting 21
- Feldenkrais Method 22
- Floatation 65
- Food Combining 22

G
- G5 Massage 66
- Galvanic Treatments 66

H
- Hair Loss 50
- Hay Diet 22
- Healing 23
- Health Resorts 23, 59
- Hellerwork 66
- Herbal Medicine 24
- Homoeopathy 24
- Hydrotherapy 25
- Hypnotherapy 26

I
- Immune System 51
- Infra-Red 67
- Ionisation 27
- Iridology 27
- Irritable Bowel Syndrome 51

J
- Joint problems 52

K
- Karwendel 67
- Kinesiology 28
- Kirlian Photography 28
- Kneipp Therapy 67

M
- Macrobiotics 28
- Magnetic Therapy 29
- Manicure 68
- Manual Lymphatic Drainage 29
- Massage 30, 68
- Meditation 30
- Megavitamin Therapy 31
- Menopause 53
- Metamorphic Technique 31
- Moor Peat Bath 68
- Mud Therapy 68

N
- Naturopathy 32
- Needle Shower 69
- Neuro Linguistic Programming 32
- Nutritional Therapy 33

O
Osteopathy	33
Osteoporosis	54

P
Panthermal	69
Paraffin Wax Baths	70
Pedicure	70
Pilates	34
Polarity Therapy	34
Premenstrual Syndrome	54
Psychotherapy	35

R
Radionics	35
Reflexology	36
Reiki	37
Relaxation Techniques	38
Rolfing	70

S
SAD	55
Salt Rub	71
Sauna	71
Sclerotherapy	71
Scottish Douche	72
Shiatsu	38
Sitz Bath	72
Spa treatments	38
Steam Bath	72
Steam Cabinet	72
Stress	55

T
T'ai-chi	39
Thai Massage	73
Thalassotherapy	73
Thrush	56
Tinnitus	57
Traditional Chinese Medicine	39
Turkish Bath	74

U
Underwater Massage	74

V
Visualisation Therapy	40
Vitamins	41

W
Waxing	74

Y
Yin and Yang	41
Yoga	41

Z
Zone Therapy	42
Zinc	44

Other Titles from Discovery Books

Healthy Breaks in Britain and Ireland
A guide to health farms and spas
by Catherine Beattie
(Published in association with the national tourist boards of England, Wales, Scotland and Northern Ireland).

The Healthy Breaks Cookbook
Easy recipes from Britain's leading health resorts
compiled by Catherine Beattie

So You Think You Need Therapy
The way to a happier life and improved relationships
by Jean Pain

So You Want to be a Therapist
by Jean Pain
(to be published in 1998)

The Really Useful Guide to Supplements
by Catherine Beattie
(to be published in 1998)

Discovery Books • 29 Hacketts Lane • Pyrford • Woking • Surrey GU22 8PP •Tel 01932 400800